HERBAL REMEDIES FOR TENDINITIS AND TENDON HEALTH

Harnessing Herbal Power For Effective Healing, Lasting Relief And Optimal Wellness

DR. CARDEN KYRIE

DISCLAIMER

The only goal of this book is informational. Every effort has been taken by the author and publisher to ensure that the information provided is accurate. But the material in this book is given "as is," without any express or implied representation, warranty, or condition as to its accuracy, completeness, or suitability for any particular purpose.

Any loss, damage, or injury resulting from using the information in this book, or from any action or decision made as a result of such use, will not be covered by the author's or publisher's liability. It is recommended that readers seek the assistance of a certified specialist for guidance specific to their situation.

The opinions and viewpoints conveyed in this book belong to the author and may not necessarily represent the official stance or policies of any specified organizations or people. Any likeness to real-life occurrences, places, or people—living or deceased—is wholly coincidental.

No specific product, service, or therapy discussed in this book is endorsed by the author or publisher. Any reference to goods or services is made only for informative reasons and is not intended as a recommendation or endorsement.

Before making any judgments or acting on any information, readers are urged to independently confirm it all. Any unfavorable effects or repercussions arising from the usage of the material included in this book are disclaimed by the author and publisher.

By using this book, you consent to absolving the publisher and author of any and all claims, obligations, or losses resulting from your use of the material in it.

I appreciate your cooperation and understanding.

TABLE OF CONTENTS

INTRODUCTION TO TENDINITIS AND TENDON HEALTH

AN OVERVIEW OF TENDINITIS

Tendinitis is a common musculoskeletal ailment that affects people of all ages and activity levels. It is characterized by inflammation of the tendons. Tendinitis can be rather severe. Tendons, the fibrous structures that link muscles to bones, are essential for stabilizing the skeletal structure and enabling joint movement. Tendinitis, the resultant inflammatory disease of these tendons, can cause discomfort, swelling, and reduced function in the affected area.

Although tendinitis can affect any portion of the body, it most frequently affects the shoulders, elbows, wrists, knees, and ankles. It frequently results from overuse of a certain joint, repeated motion, or poor biomechanics during physical activity. Effective tendinitis prevention and treatment depend on an understanding of the underlying mechanisms and causes of the illness.

TENDON HEALTH IS IMPORTANT

It is impossible to overestimate the significance of tendon health because these fibrous structures are essential to the musculoskeletal system's entire functionality. Tendons serve as the link between the muscles and the bones, transferring the force produced by a muscle contraction into motion. Ankle elasticity, joint function, and general physical performance all depend on the health and integrity of tendons.

Tendon health is especially important in the context of sports and physical activity when the musculoskeletal system is under increased stress. Due to the repeated strains exerted on particular joints and tendons, athletes and those involved in intensive activities are especially prone to tendinitis. Thus, maintaining optimal physical performance and lowering the risk of injury depends heavily on techniques for controlling and preventing tendinitis.

Beyond the realm of sports, tendinitis can also impact people in their everyday lives, particularly those who perform repetitive tasks at work or engage in activities that require extended durations of joint activity. Reduced productivity, worse quality of life, and possibly long-term effects if treatment is not received are all effects of tendinitis.

To shed light on the nature, causes, and prevalence of tendinitis, this introduction attempts to give a general overview of the condition. It also highlights the vital role that tendon health plays in preserving general musculoskeletal health, emphasizing the significance of taking preventative and remedial action to avoid and treat tendinitis in people with a variety of lifestyles and activity levels.

CHAPTER ONE

KNOWLEDGE ABOUT TENDINITIS

TENDINITIS: DEFINITION AND CAUSES

The thick fibrous cord that connects muscle to bone is called a tendon, and tendinitis, or tendinitis, is a medical ailment marked by inflammation of the tendon. Usually brought on by overuse, trauma, or aging, this inflammation causes pain and discomfort in the affected area. Though it can affect any tendon in the body, the shoulders, elbows, wrists, knees, and heels are the most frequently affected? If left untreated, the illness, which usually appears gradually, can become a chronic problem.

Tendinitis develops as a result of several circumstances. Inflammation can result from overuse or repetitive motions, such as those required in some sports or jobs, which can strain the tendons. Tendinitis can also be brought on by unexpected trauma or injury. Tendon deterioration due to aging may also play a role since tendons lose some of their flexibility and become more vulnerable to damage. In certain instances, tendinitis risk may be elevated by underlying medical disorders, such as diabetes or rheumatoid arthritis.

TENDINITIS TYPES

Tendinitis comes in various forms, each linked to certain tendons and body parts that are impacted. Acute tendinitis is the term for an abrupt and severe tendon inflammation that frequently follows a particular trauma or injury. The afflicted area usually experiences severe pain, swelling, and tenderness when this kind of tendinitis occurs. Conversely, chronic tendinitis is a condition that worsens over time as a result of repeated strain on the tendon, causing discomfort that lasts longer. Although the symptoms of chronic tendinitis may not be as severe, they can persist for a long time, thus it's crucial to treat the illness to avoid developing worsening consequences.

TYPICAL SYMPTOMS

Pain and discomfort in the affected area, particularly when movement or when pressure is applied, are common signs of tendinitis. There may also be warmth and swelling surrounding the tendon, and in certain situations, there may be less range of motion. Depending on the particular tendon impacted and the degree of inflammation, tendinitis can present with a variety of symptoms. To provide an accurate diagnosis and suitable treatment, it is imperative to distinguish tendinitis from other disorders that present with similar symptoms, such as bursitis or arthritis.

FACTORS AT RISK FOR TENDINITIS

The probability of tendinitis is increased by certain risk factors. Overuse and strain on the tendons can result from repetitive motions or activities, especially in sports or jobs requiring regular use of certain muscle groups. Inadequate technique and inadequate training during physical exercises could also be contributing factors.

Age plays a big role because as people age, their tendons lose some of their flexibility and become more prone to damage. Obesity, diabetes, and rheumatoid arthritis are a few illnesses that can raise the risk of tendinitis. An increased incidence of tendinitis has also been associated with smoking and the use of specific drugs, including corticosteroids and fluoroquinolone antibiotics.

Tendinitis is a common ailment that is typified by tendon inflammation, frequently brought on by age, injury, or overuse. Acute tendinitis is characterized by rapid, severe symptoms, while chronic tendinitis develops gradually over time. Pain, soreness, edema, and decreased range of motion are typical symptoms. Tendinitis develops as a result of several risk factors, such as age, underlying medical disorders, and repetitive activities. To effectively manage tendinitis and avoid long-term consequences, prompt diagnosis and intervention are crucial.

CHAPTER TWO

TENDON ANATOMY

TENDON STRUCTURE

Tendon structure is an intricate configuration of connective tissue that is essential to the function of the musculoskeletal system. Tendons are bands of fibrous tissue, mostly made of collagen, and they have a hierarchical structure that gives these structures strength and flexibility. Tendons, which connect muscles to bones by resembling cords, are structures that, when viewed at a macroscopic level, let the skeletal framework absorb the mechanical stresses produced during muscle contraction.

Collagen fibers are arranged in a parallel pattern, creating a hierarchical structure that spans from the macroscopic to the microscopic level and offers resilience and tensile strength to withstand the stresses brought on by movement.

TENDON FUNCTION

Tendons play an important functional role in the body's biomechanical apparatus. Their major job is to transfer the contractile forces produced by muscles to bones so that movements can be carried out and joints can remain stable. To enable coordinated and effective movement, tendon structures serve as a bridge, facilitating the smooth passage of force from contracting muscle fibers to the skeletal elements. Tendons' mechanical characteristics, like their strength and elasticity, are precisely calibrated to match the demands of different types of physical activity.

TENDON FUNCTIONS IN THE BODY

Recognizing tendons' function in the musculoskeletal system is essential to understanding how tendons function in the body. Joint movement is the outcome of a muscle's contraction, which produces a force that travels from the muscle to the bone via a tendon. It is possible to perform both simple and sophisticated movements with this coordinated action, from the simple act of walking to the precise dexterity needed for tasks like typing or playing an instrument. Tendons provide a structural foundation for preserving appropriate anatomical alignment and inhibit excessive movement, which helps to preserve joint stability.

THE VALUE OF KEEPING TENDONS HEALTHY

One cannot stress how crucial it is to keep tendons in good condition because they are essential to general mobility and functionality. Tendon injuries, including strains and ruptures, can seriously hinder a person's capacity to carry out everyday tasks and exercise. Age, excessive use, and poor training are some of the variables that might cause tendon degeneration and raise the risk of injury. Maintaining the health of tendons requires a proper diet, consistent exercise, and enough sleep. Furthermore, correcting biomechanical abnormalities and employing the right approaches when exercising will help reduce the chance of tendon-related problems.

Tendons are essential to the musculoskeletal system's structural and functional integrity. The complex arrangement of these bones, which is engineered to endure mechanical strains, facilitates the effective transfer of force produced by muscles to bones. Comprehending the role of tendons in the body highlights their importance in promoting mobility and preserving joint stability. Sustaining robust tendons is critical for general health, underscoring the necessity of preventive actions and lifestyle decisions that support good tendon function and resilience.

CHAPTER THREE

HERBAL TENDINITIS REMEDIES

AN OVERVIEW OF HERBAL MEDICINE

Phytotherapy, another name for herbal medicine, is a holistic approach to healing that uses plants and plant-derived chemicals to treat a range of illnesses. Traditional medicinal systems around the world, including Ayurveda,

Traditional Chinese Medicine (TCM), and Native American medicine, have included this age-old practice as a crucial component. Herbal treatments are prized for their ability to treat the root causes of health problems in addition to their symptoms. Herbal therapy provides a variety of possibilities for managing inflammation and accelerating the healing process in the setting of tendinitis.

STANDARDS FOR SELECTING HERBAL TREATMENTS

Various factors can help in the selection process while looking for herbal remedies for tendinitis. First and foremost, extensive research is needed to determine the herbs' safety and effectiveness. Selecting herbs that have a track record of traditional usage and scientific proof of their anti-inflammatory and restorative effects is crucial. The person's overall health and medical history should also be considered, as some plants may interfere with prescription drugs or pre-existing diseases.

HERBS THAT REDUCE INFLAMMATION IN TENDINITIS

Since inflammation is a major cause of the pain and discomfort that tendinitis causes, anti-inflammatory medicines are essential for addressing this ailment. One such herb is turmeric (Curcuma longa), whose active ingredient, curcumin, is known for its strong anti-inflammatory qualities. In Ayurvedic medicine, this herbal cure has been used for generations to ease pain and reduce inflammation. You can take turmeric in several ways, including drinks, capsules, and meals.

GINGER

The plant ginger, or Zingiber officinale, is renowned for its ability to reduce inflammation. It has bioactive ingredients like gingerol, which has been demonstrated to prevent the body from producing inflammatory chemicals. You can drink ginger tea, eat it raw, or take it as a supplement. Due to its adaptability, this herb can be easily included in one's daily routine as it adds flavor and accessibility to a wide range of foods.

BOSWELLIA

Indian frankincense, or Boswellia (Boswellia serrata), is well known for its analgesic and anti-inflammatory qualities. Studies have been conducted on the potential of boswellic acids, the active ingredients in boswellia, to reduce inflammation and promote joint health. Supplements containing Boswellia come in a variety of formats, such as capsules and topical treatments.

Finally, herbal treatments provide a comprehensive and all-natural way to treat tendinitis. Herbs with anti-inflammatory properties that have demonstrated the potential to reduce symptoms and accelerate the healing process include turmeric, ginger, and boswellia. But before adding herbal therapies to a treatment plan, it is important to speak with a healthcare provider, particularly if there are any co-occurring medical issues or drugs. With careful thought and well-informed decision-making, the incorporation of herbal medicine into the overall therapy of tendinitis should be tackled.

CHAPTER FOUR

HERBAL REMEDIES FOR PAIN

WILLOW BARK

Willow bark's ability to relieve pain has long been known, having been used by ancient societies. Salicin, the main ingredient in willow bark, has analgesic and anti-inflammatory properties and is comparable to aspirin. Willow bark has been used to treat a variety of pains, such as headaches, aches in the muscles, and sore joints. Because of its capacity to control inflammation, it is a natural option for people looking for herbal pain relievers.

ARNICA

The plant Arnica montana is the source of the well-known anti-inflammatory herb Arnica. Arnica is a popular ingredient in topical formulations like lotions and ointments because of its ability to lessen swelling and ease pain from sprains, bruises, and sore muscles.

The plant is a popular option for external applications in the field of herbal pain therapy because of its anti-inflammatory properties, which are attributed to its active components, including helenalin.

HERBS THAT PROMOTE BETTER BLOOD FLOW

Herbs that promote better circulation are essential for relieving pain because they increase blood flow to the afflicted areas. The Ginkgo biloba plant, which yields leaves, is well-known for its vasodilatory properties, which aid in improving circulation. This herb may help control pain related to poor blood circulation since it is thought to improve the supply of nutrients and oxygen to tissues. Supplements containing ginkgo biloba are frequently taken into account for their ability to promote general vascular health.

CAYENNE

The chemical recognized for its analgesic effects, capsaicin, is found in cayenne, which is derived from spicy chili peppers. Because of its capacity to desensitize nerve receptors and lessen the experience of pain, cayenne has long been used topically. Creams or ointments containing cayenne administered topically may provide relief from arthritic pain and neuropathic discomfort. The heat effect that cayenne produces may enhance blood flow, which bolsters its potential as an analgesic.

HERBAL MIXTURES FOR HEALTHY TENDONS

Herbal remedies designed specifically to support the health of the tendon can offer a comprehensive strategy for managing pain and enhancing general well-being. Herbal mixtures that include ginger, Boswellia, and turmeric are known to have anti-inflammatory qualities. These mixtures are designed to lessen inflammation and aid in tendon recovery. Particularly, turmeric has the powerful anti-inflammatory component curcumin, and boswellia has long been used to relieve pain in the joints and tendons. Because of its anti-inflammatory and antioxidant qualities, ginger enhances the benefits of these herbs, making herbal combos a worthwhile option for anyone looking for all-around tendon health assistance. By including these herbs in one's wellness regimen, one may help preserve and restore the health of their tendons and provide a natural option for those seeking to control pain and enhance joint function in general.

CHAPTER FIVE

TENDON NUTRITIONAL SUPPORT

NUTRITION'S SIGNIFICANCE FOR TENDON HEALTH

The fibrous structures that join muscles to bones are called tendons, and their health is greatly influenced by diet. Sufficient dietary intake is necessary for tendon upkeep, repair, and general health. It is impossible to exaggerate the significance of a good diet for tendon health because it directly affects the body's capacity to heal from wounds, fend against degeneration, and maintain peak performance.

FOODS FOR MAINTAINING AND REPAIRING TENDONS

Eating foods that aid in tendon maintenance and healing is essential for maintaining tendon health. These foods ought to be high in nutrients that support the production of collagen, an essential step for the strength and flexibility of tendons. The primary structural protein in tendons, collagen, needs particular nutrients to be produced and repaired. For tendons to remain intact and be able to tolerate mechanical stress, it is essential to make sure they are getting enough of these nutrients.

FATTY ACIDS OMEGA-3

Because of their ability to reduce inflammation, omega-3 fatty acids are essential for the health of tendons. Omega-3 fatty acids, which are present in fatty fish like salmon, mackerel, and flaxseeds, can help lessen tendon inflammation and provide an environment that is more conducive to healing. Including these foods in the diet helps maintain the general anti-inflammatory balance that is essential for the health of the tendons.

FOODS HIGH IN VITAMIN C

Strong antioxidant vitamin C is necessary for the production of collagen and is also vital for the integrity of tendons. Vitamin C-rich foods including bell peppers, strawberries, and citrus fruits can help maintain and repair tendon structures. By adding these foods to the diet, one can support the development of collagen, which strengthens and resilient tendons.

RICH IN ZINC AND COPPER FOODS

Trace minerals like zinc and copper are important for the synthesis and maturation of collagen. Zinc-rich foods include shellfish, organ meats, and whole grains; copper-rich foods include nuts, seeds, and lean meats. By supporting the biochemical processes involved in tendon repair, ensuring an appropriate intake of these minerals eventually helps to maintain the health of the tendon.

SUPPLEMENTS MADE OF HERBS FOR TENDON HEALTH

Supplemental herbal remedies may also be advantageous for tendon health. Curcumin and Boswellia serrata are examples of substances with anti-inflammatory qualities that may help reduce tendon-related pain. These supplements offer an alternate or supplementary strategy to conventional dietary assistance for tendon health, while they should still be used carefully and ideally under a doctor's supervision.

Sustaining optimal tendon health requires putting nutrition first. A diet high in zinc, copper, vitamin C, omega-3 fatty acids, and possibly even some herbal supplements can offer complete support for tendon maintenance and repair. This all-encompassing nutritional approach not only speeds up the healing process following tendon injuries but also enhances the durability and functionality of these essential connective tissues over the long run.

CHAPTER SIX

ADJUSTMENTS TO LIFESTYLE FOR TENDON HEALTH

EXERCISE'S SIGNIFICANCE FOR TENDON HEALTH

Exercise is essential for preserving and enhancing the health of tendons. An essential part of the musculoskeletal system is tendon connections, which link muscles to bones. Frequent exercise improves the strength, flexibility, and resilience of tendons, which benefits their general health. Exercises that combine strengthening and stretching are especially advantageous for the health of tendons.

EXERCISES TO STRETCH AND STRENGTHEN

Stretching activities help tendons become more flexible, which increases their range of motion and lowers the chance of damage. Before engaging in more demanding activities, dynamic stretches like arm circles and leg swings can help warm up the muscles and tendons. Furthermore, over time, static stretches—in which the muscle is maintained in an extended position—promote greater flexibility.

Exercises aimed at strengthening tendons are crucial for increasing their resiliency. Tendon strength is developed through resistance training, which includes exercises using resistance bands and weightlifting. Tendon health and durability are enhanced by gradually increasing the resistance and intensity of these activities.

TENDON HEALTH WITH YOGA

Another exercise that can make a big difference in tendon health is yoga. Yoga's deliberate motions stretches, and mindfulness practices all work together to build strength, balance, and flexibility. Some yoga poses target tendons specifically to help with their overall health and conditioning.

PARTICULAR EXERCISES FOR VARIOUS TENDONS

For a thorough approach to tendon health, it is necessary to modify activities to target particular tendons. Each tendon in the body has its specific purpose and needs. For instance, calf rises and heel drops are workouts that target the Achilles tendon, whereas shoulder-strengthening exercises are activities that target the rotator cuff. A focused exercise program guarantees that every tendon gets the care it needs for optimum health.

TENDON HEALTH AND ERGONOMICS

Maintaining tendon health is greatly aided by ergonomics, particularly when it comes to daily activities and work-related responsibilities. Whether at work or during leisure activities, good ergonomics lessens the strain on tendons. To avoid overuse and tiredness, this entails adopting ergonomic equipment, keeping proper posture, and taking regular pauses.

STRATEGIES FOR REST AND RECUPERATION

Both recuperation and rest are essential parts of a comprehensive strategy for tendon health. Tendons can heal from the strains of everyday activity and exercise when they get enough sleep. Chronic diseases and overuse injuries can result from inadequate sleep. Promoting tendon repair requires including rest days into a workout regimen and placing a high priority on getting enough sleep.

A holistic lifestyle approach to supporting tendon health combines stretching, strengthening activities, yoga, specialized exercises for certain tendons, ergonomic habits, and enough rest and recuperation. By incorporating these components into daily life, tendons are strengthened, flexible, and resilient, which benefits the musculoskeletal system as a whole.

CHAPTER SIX

COMBINING CONVENTIONAL TREATMENTS WITH HERBAL REMEDIES

WORKING TOGETHER WITH HEALTHCARE EXPERTS

People looking for alternative medicines and healthcare experts must work together to integrate herbal remedies with conventional treatments. To guarantee a thorough understanding of a patient's health profile, it is imperative to establish open communication and transparency regarding the usage of herbal supplements. Healthcare professionals, such as physicians, nurses, and pharmacists, can provide insightful information on possible interactions between prescription drugs and herbal treatments, assisting in the prevention of side effects and improving treatment results.

Patients are encouraged to actively participate in decisions about herbal remedies with their healthcare team by using this collaborative paradigm. Experts can offer their knowledge in evaluating the efficacy of herbal remedies based on scientific evidence, taking into account elements like dose, purity, and possible adverse effects. Patients can gain from a more holistic approach to their care that combines both conventional and herbal therapies by creating an atmosphere of shared decision-making.

COMBINING HERBAL REMEDIES WITH CONVENTIONAL MEDICATION

Acknowledging the advantages and disadvantages of both approaches is necessary when combining herbal remedies with conventional medication. Conventional medicine, which is supported by extensive scientific research, frequently uses standardized medications with proven safety and efficacy profiles. Herbal treatments, on the other hand, are based on age-old methods and may provide supplementary or substitute treatments, especially when it comes to treating chronic illnesses or enhancing general health.

When it comes to helping patients include herbal treatments in their treatment regimens, healthcare experts can be extremely helpful. This entails determining if herbal supplements and prescription drugs mix well, analyzing any potential benefits, and keeping an eye out for any negative side effects. In turn, patients gain from a more individualized and comprehensive approach to healthcare that takes into account their particular needs and makes use of the combined knowledge of herbal and traditional medicine.

POSSIBLE DANGERS AND THINGS TO THINK ABOUT

Even while combining herbal medicines with conventional treatments may have advantages, there may be hazards that should be recognized and addressed. A major worry is the potential for herb-drug interactions, in which taking herbal supplements could affect how well prescription drugs are absorbed, metabolized, or excreted. Healthcare practitioners must be informed by patients about the usage of herbal supplements so they can recognize and handle any potential interactions that can reduce the efficacy of treatment.

Furthermore, there are questions regarding standardization and safety because there can be wide variations in the quality and purity of herbal products. Patients should be made aware of the value of purchasing herbal treatments from reliable suppliers and the necessity of quality assurance procedures. Furthermore, there's a chance that certain herbal therapies come with unintentional dangers, like allergic responses or conflicts with certain medical conditions.

A cooperative and knowledgeable approach is needed to successfully include herbal therapies with conventional treatments. Both patients and healthcare providers need to be transparent about the advantages and disadvantages of mixing traditional and herbal medicine. People can better navigate this integrative method and ensure a thorough and well-balanced approach to healthcare by encouraging a collaborative decision-making process.

CHAPTER SEVEN

CASE STUDIES AND TRIUMPHANT NARRATIVES

ACTUAL HERBAL MEDICINE EXPERIENCES

Herbal medicine has a lengthy history of being woven into human history, providing a legacy of therapeutic techniques that have been passed down through the ages. True stories of healing and resiliency through the use of herbal treatments have frequently been included in the complex mix of traditional knowledge and contemporary medicine. People from a variety of backgrounds have shared their experiences, attesting to the herbs' transformational ability in treating a range of health issues.

These first-hand narratives frequently underscore the holistic character of herbal treatments, stressing not only their physiological advantages but also their positive effects on mental and emotional health. These accounts highlight the diverse range of benefits that herbal therapies can provide those looking for complementary and alternative medicine, from improving immune system function to relieving chronic pain.

STORIES OF SUCCESSFUL TENDON RECOVERY

Due to tendon injuries' propensity for a protracted healing period, people have been looking for creative rehabilitation strategies. Success stories show up amid these difficulties as rays of hope and motivation. These stories often highlight the human body's tenacity and the effectiveness of all-encompassing tendon rehabilitation techniques.

Success stories involving tendon recovery typically result from a confluence of circumstances, such as individualized rehabilitation regimens, following medical recommendations, and occasionally including complementary therapies like herbal remedies. These stories show the value of mental toughness and an optimistic outlook in overcoming the difficult process of tendon rehabilitation in addition to physical recovery.

TEACHINGS LESSONS ACQUIRED FROM CASE STUDIES

Case studies are incredibly useful sources of information because they shed light on the complexities of different illnesses and how to treat them. The knowledge gained from these in-depth analyses greatly advances medicine by enabling researchers and practitioners to improve patient outcomes and treatment strategies.

A recurrent element in the analysis of case studies is the significance of personalized healthcare. The variety of medical issues necessitates individualized treatments that take into account each patient's particular situation. Furthermore, case studies frequently highlight the value of a multidisciplinary approach, in which cooperation between medical specialists from various specialties improves the comprehensiveness of care.

TENDON HEALTH EMPOWERING READERS

Giving people the tools they need to take charge of their tendon health entails raising awareness, encouraging preventive care, and sharing knowledge. The use of herbal medicines and other holistic approaches in real-life success stories is essential in motivating readers to give their tendon health priority.

Readers are empowered to make informed lifestyle decisions when educational campaigns emphasize common risk factors for injuries, the architecture of tendons, and preventive techniques. People are better able to form behaviors that extend the life and elasticity of their tendons when they comprehend the connections between exercise, diet, and general health. Encouraging readers to take an active role in their tendon health goes beyond therapy; it's a commitment to overall health and a proactive approach to keeping a strong musculoskeletal system.

CHAPTER EIGHT

SECTION ON RECIPES

RECIPES FOR HERBAL REMEDIES

Using the medicinal qualities of several plants to enhance health and well-being, herbal remedies have long been a mainstay of conventional medicine. These recipes frequently call for the deft blending of many herbs to produce powerful mixtures that effectively treat a variety of illnesses. Herbal treatments offer a comprehensive method of healing that draws on the innate strength of plants, whether they are used to ease digestive problems, relieve the symptoms of a common cold, or encourage relaxation.

HERBAL SOAKS

Traditionally, the medicinal powers of herbs have been utilized externally through the use of herbal poultices. Traditionally, a poultice is made by combining moist, soft herbs into a mass and applying it directly to the skin. By using this technique, the beneficial elements of the herbs are absorbed by the skin, relieving ailments including inflammation, discomfort in the muscles, and skin irritations. Herbal poultices are a flexible and individualized form of topical herbal treatment since they may be customized to target particular issues.

TINCTURES AND INFUSIONS

These herbal preparations in liquid form are meant to extract and concentrate the therapeutic qualities of plants. Herbs are steeped in glycerin or alcohol to extract the active ingredients gradually, as in tinctures. But infusions, which are made similarly to tea, are made by steeping herbs in hot water. Strong liquid extracts with easy-to-consume medicinal effects are produced by both procedures. While infusions offer a milder approach to experiencing the flavors and therapeutic properties of herbs, tinctures are frequently chosen due to their concentrated nature and extended shelf life.

HERBAL SALVES

Using oils or beeswax and herbs, herbal salves are applied preparations that provide a calming, nourishing balm. These salves are frequently applied to skin ailments such as burns, wounds, and dry skin. The herbal salve is made by infusing a few chosen herbs into a carrier oil, which is then combined with beeswax to harden the concoction into the consistency of a salve. Applying the final product directly to the skin will enable the herbal ingredients to be absorbed and provide targeted relief. Herbal salves are a great example of how adaptable herbs are for supporting skin health and offering specific help for a range of dermatological issues.

The realm of herbal treatments comprises a wide range of preparations, each possessing distinct advantages and uses.

www.ingramcontent.com/pod-product-compliance
Lightning Source LLC
Chambersburg PA
CBHW060848260726
48661CB00002B/670